Najla BAHLOUL
Mariem AYADI

Exogenous lipid pneumonias

Najla BAHLOUL
Mariem AYADI

Exogenous lipid pneumonias

Imprint
Any brand names and product names mentioned in this book are subject to trademark, brand or patent protection and are trademarks or registered trademarks of their respective holders. The use of brand names, product names, common names, trade names, product descriptions etc. even without a particular marking in this work is in no way to be construed to mean that such names may be regarded as unrestricted in respect of trademark and brand protection legislation and could thus be used by anyone.

Cover image: www.ingimage.com

This book is a translation from the original published under ISBN 978-620-6-71835-2.

Publisher:
Sciencia Scripts
is a trademark of
Dodo Books Indian Ocean Ltd. and OmniScriptum S.R.L publishing group

120 High Road, East Finchley, London, N2 9ED, United Kingdom
Str. Armeneasca 28/1, office 1, Chisinau MD-2012, Republic of Moldova, Europe
Printed at: see last page
ISBN: 978-620-7-95501-5

Introduction

Lipid pneumonia is a rare condition resulting from an accumulation of lipids in the alveoli of the lungs. These fatty compounds may be of animal, vegetable or mineral origin (1, 2).

Lipid pneumonia may be endogenous (caused by lipids in lung tissue metabolised by obstructive or inflammatory processes) or exogenous (caused by inhalation or aspiration of oily substances).

Exogenous lipid pneumonia (ELP) can be acute or chronic (3). Acute ELP occurs when a large quantity of lipid substance is aspirated, whereas chronic exogenous lipoid pneumonia occurs after repeated episodes of aspiration or inhalation of lipids over a prolonged period (3).

It may be under-diagnosed because it is confused with other conditions such as bacterial pneumonia, lung tumour, tuberculosis or organised pneumonia, given its non-specific presentation and the absence of exposure (4).

The radiological lesions of exogenous lipid pneumonia are not specific and vary from patient to patient and from acute to chronic (5).

Diagnosis is based on anatomopathological data. However, it can be confirmed without recourse to invasive procedures by a good knowledge of the causes and manifestations of this condition, when the history, exposure, clinical, radiological and cytological findings are concordant.

There are currently no specific recommendations for the treatment of this disease.

However, it is essential to stop exposure to the oily substances involved. Corticosteroid therapy may be useful, depending on the severity of the pneumonia.

Mild cases develop favourably within a few weeks, while more severe cases may progress to pulmonary fibrosis and persistent respiratory symptoms (6).

Ethiopathogeny

1. Ethiopathogeny

1.1. Age

The average age of patients varies between 45 and 68.5 years (Table I).

Table I Average age of patients with PLE

Series	Years	Number of cases	Average age
Acharya et al (7)	2021	3	52 years old
Aliaga et al (8)	2017	3	68 years old
Gondouin et al (9)	1996	44	62 years old
Han et al (10)	2016	3	45 years old
Osman et al (11)	2018	4	68.5 years old
Samhouri et al (12)	2021	34	71 years old

1.2. Gender

The data in the literature are divergent. A number of authors suggest a male predominance. Other publications tend to favour a female predominance (Table II).

Table II Breakdown by gender

Series	Years	Number of cases	Men	Woman
Acharya et al (7)	2021	3	2	1
Aliaga et al (8)	2017	3	2	1
Gondouin et al (9)	1996	44	20	24
Han et al (10)	2016	3	0	3
Osman et al (11)	2018	4	2	2
Samhouri et al (12)	2021	34	15	18

1.3. Pathophysiology

The primum movens is the presence of an oily substance aspirated or inhaled into the pulmonary alveoli, which will be phagocytised by macrophages (13).

After their death, the macrophages release the oil, leading to a granulomatous giant cell inflammatory reaction and fibrosis (13).

Clinical study

2. Clinical study

2.1. Circumstances of discovery

2.1.1. Accidental discovery

Lipid pneumonia may be discovered by chance during a chest X-ray performed as part of a preoperative check-up (14) (Table III).

Patients are often asymptomatic despite extensive radiological images discovered incidentally on routine chest X-rays (5).

Table III Cases of incidental exogenous lipid pneumonia

Series	Year	Gender	Design
M. Doubková et al (14)	2013	Woman	Pre-operative assessment
Nakashima S et al (15)	2015	Men	Routine checks
Ohwada et al (16)	2002	Men	Routine checks

2.1.2. Symptomatic forms (Table IV)

Typical symptoms of acute ELP include cough, dyspnoea and fever.

Chronic ELP may be accompanied by cough and dyspnoea. Fever, weight loss and chest pain are less common. Sputum and chest pain are not uncommon. Haemoptysis is exceptional (3).

Table IVFunctional signs in PLE

Series	Acharya et al (7)	Gondouin et al (9)	Han et al (10)
Dyspnoea	100%	50%	100%
Cough	100%	64%	100%
Sputum	100%	28%	100%
Haemoptysis	0%	13%	0%
Chest pain	0%	21%	100%
Fever	100%	39%	0%
Weight loss	33,33%	34%	0%

Thoracic imaging

3. Thoracic imaging

3.1. CT scan technique

Thoracic computed tomography (CT) is an essential examination for diagnosing exogenous lipid pneumonia. It is performed using a high-resolution technique with thin-slice reconstruction, without injection of contrast medium to assess the lung parenchyma and then with injection of contrast medium to assess the mediastinal structures (2).

The CT scan is generally performed in the inspiratory phase, although it is sometimes necessary to add slices in the expiratory phase to look for air trapping.

3.2. Scannographic aspects of acute ELP

Acute PLE may take the form of areas of consolidation or bilateral ground-glass opacities in the middle and lower lobes (3).

A CT scan may reveal areas of fat density, which may however be masked by a simultaneous inflammatory process (3).

3.3. Scannographic aspects of chronic PLE

The radiological lesions are multiple and often associated. None of these aspects constitutes a specific radiological feature of PLE (Table V) (5).

The most common radiological abnormality is parenchymal condensation. This is an area of systematised or non-systematised pulmonary parenchymal overdensity, obliterating the pulmonary vessels.

However, ground-glass images are frequently described in series. This is a diffuse or focal increase in the density of the lung parenchyma, without blurring of the pulmonary vessel contours, and reflects partial filling of the alveolar lumina and/or thickening of the alveolar partitions (17).

The crazy paving appearance is characterised by a diffuse or disseminated ground-glass opacity with superimposed interlobular and intra-lobular interstitial thickening on high-resolution CT. This appearance, which is classically suggestive of alveolar proteinosis, has been reported in PLE (Figure 1) (18).

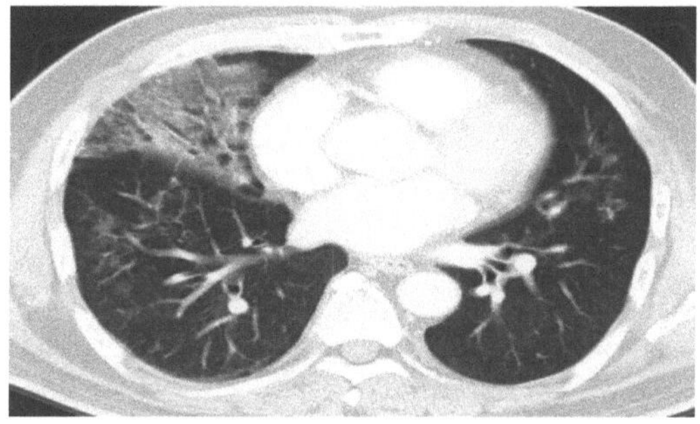

Figure 1: Crazy paving in the middle lobe (18)

PLE can present as a pulmonary nodule, which places it in the differential diagnosis of lung cancer (Figure 2) (19, 20)..

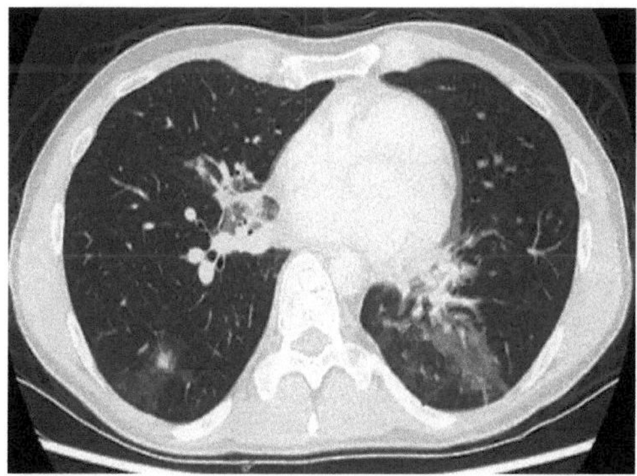

Figure 2: Nodule surrounded by a ground-glass opacity in the right lower lobe and consolidation in the left lower lobe (20)

The most characteristic lesion of PLE is the presence of areas with a negative fat attenuation value, between -30 HU and -150 HU, measured at the level of consolidations or nodules, with or without a peripheral fibrous reaction (2).

Table VScannographic aspects of PLE

	Frosted glass	Parenchymal condensation	Crazy paving	Nodule	Adenopathy
Cozzi et al (2)	100%	80%	60%	20%	50%
Samhouri et al (12)	82,35%	64,7%	26,47%	61,76%	8,82%
Marchiori et al (21)	37,7%	86,6%	20,7%	22,6%	0%

Other radiological abnormalities may be seen, including pneumatoceles (Figure 3 and 4), excavated nodules or abscesses (Figure 5 and 6), pneumomediastinum, pneumothorax and pleural effusions (1, 13).

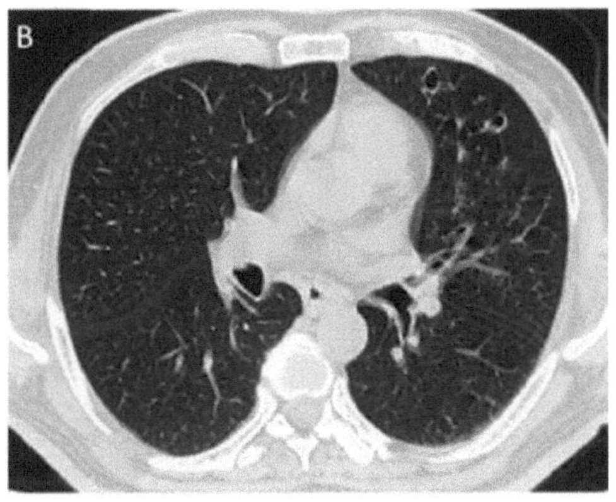

Figure 3: Pneumatoceles of the left upper lobe (1)

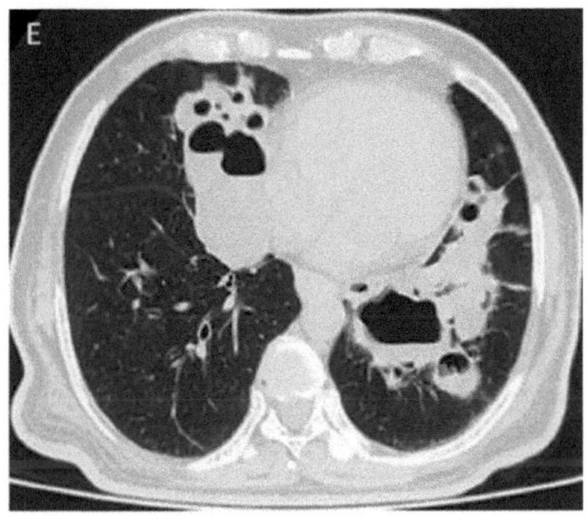

Figure 4: Bilateral condensations with pneumatoceles containing hydroaerobic levels (1)

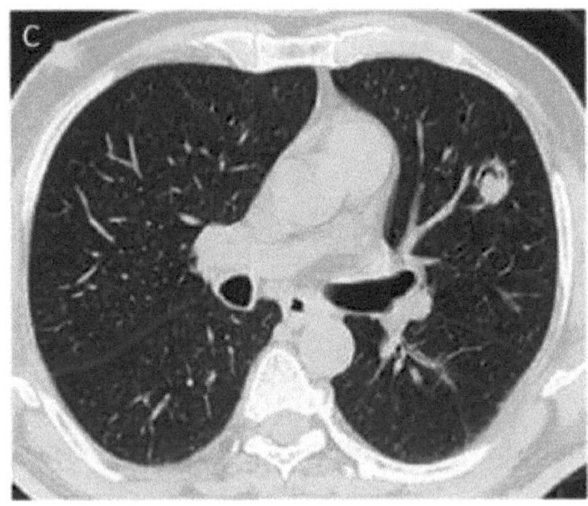

Figure 5: Excavated nodule in the left upper lobe (1)

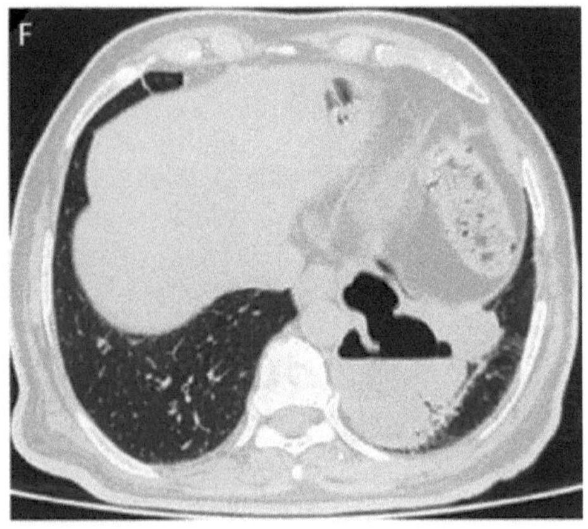

Figure 6: Abscessed cavity in the left lower lobe (1)

The angiogram sign can be found and consists of an enhancement of the normal vascular architecture within a parenchymal condensation on a CT scan performed with injection of contrast medium. This sign is non-specific for PLE (22).

The topography of these lesions is a fundamental diagnostic criterion because the disease is clearly predominant in the declinal regions (lower lobes, middle lobe, lingula) (23)..

According to a review of the literature by Guo et al, PLE is more likely to occur in the middle and lower lobes bilaterally (24).

Distribution is essentially peribronchovascular (3).

Means of diagnostic confirmation

4. Means of confirming the diagnosis of PLE (Table VI)

The test of choice for confirmatory diagnosis is bronchioloalveolar lavage (BAL) with biopsies (7). BAL may reveal a cloudy or whitish fluid with fat droplets visible to the naked eye on the surface. Transparietal biopsy under CT scan may be diagnostic and in some cases surgical biopsy may be necessary (Figure 7) (20, 25).

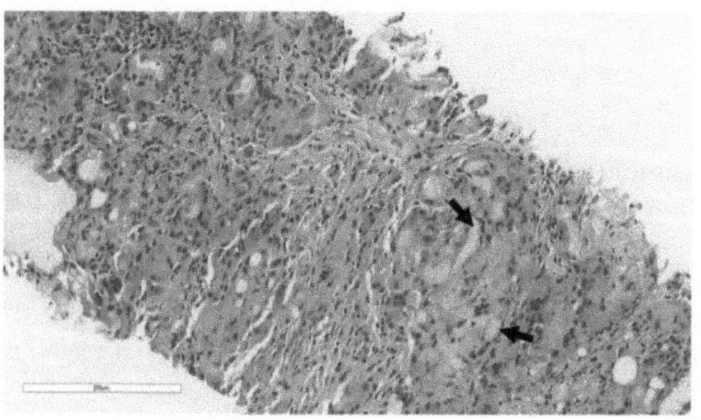

Figure 7: Lung biopsy showing an amorphous acellular substance with a giant cell reaction to a foreign body (20).

Histological specimens cannot be preserved in paraffin, as the lipids are dissolved by xylol and other substances used during processing (5). The different characteristics of oils can be detected by histochemical reactions on Sudan IV and Oil red O stain (26).

Oil Red O (Solvent Red 27 or Sudan Red 5B) is a lysochromic (fat-soluble) diazo dye used for staining triglycerides and neutral lipids in frozen tissue sections or unfixed (air-dried) cytology slides (smears and/or touch preparations) (27). Oil Red O staining is used to identify lipid-laden macrophages (28). Oil Red O-positive macrophages are numerous in cases of lipid pneumonia (Figure 8).

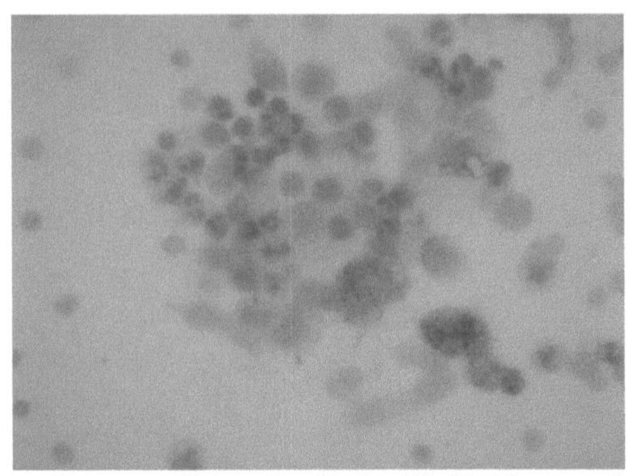

Figure 8: Presence of macrophages loaded with lipid vacuoles (staining: Oil red O x 400)

PLE can be discovered post mortem in a series of cases reported by Rana et al. (26).

Table VI Different means of confirmation in ELPs

	LBA	Bronchial biopsy	Transparietal biopsy	Surgical biopsy	Autopsy
Gondouin et al (9)	68,18%	15,9%	2,27%	13,63%	0%
Samhouri et al (12)	8,82%	44,11%	8,82%	17,64%	0%
Marchiori et al (21)	77,35%	0%	0%	16,98%	5,66%

Aetiological assessment

5. Etiologies and contributing factors

The substance most frequently inhaled by patients was mineral oil (29). It may inhibit the cough reflex and ciliary motility, thereby facilitating inhalation (16).

Among the most incriminated mineral oils are oil-based laxatives for the treatment of constipation (paraffin oil) (30), nasal decongestants for chronic nasopharyngeal diseases (11), vaping (31), fish oil capsules (32), fire-breathing lung oil (33).

Vegetable oils have also been described as responsible for PLE, such as oil extraction; this involves putting a tablespoon of oil (coconut, sesame or sunflower oil) in the mouth and swishing it around for around 20 minutes in the morning (34). Animal oils are also incriminated but less frequently, causing intense inflammation and fibrosis depending on the free fatty acid content (35).

Sometimes more than one substance was identified. Most patients had been using the substance(s) in question for years or even decades (Table VII) (12).

Table VII Other substances reported in the literature that can cause PLE

- Insecticide (isoparaffin) (36)
- Inhalation of vaporised paraffin from candles (37)
- Inhalation of herbicide (38)
- Use of lip gloss or lip balm (39)
- Vaseline used in the care of tracheotomy patients (40)
- Occupational exposure to engine oils (22)
- Exposure to solvent aerosols (41)
- Smoking lipid-based products with drugs as a preservation technique (42)
- Gavage of infants with animal fats (clarified butter in Saudi Arabia) (43)
- Using Vicks VapoRub® (44)
- Milk consumption (15)

Impaired swallowing due to anatomical or functional abnormalities of the pharynx and oesophagus (hiatal hernia, gastro-oesophageal reflux, megaesophagus, Zenker's diverticulum, achalasia) can be a factor favouring aspiration, as can neuromuscular diseases affecting pharyngeal motility or the cough reflex, psychiatric disorders and episodes of loss of consciousness (5, 13).

Differential diagnosis

6. Differential diagnosis

6.1. Hamartomas

Hamartomas are the most common benign tumours of the lung. They appear as fat-containing lesions on CT scan, sometimes with calcifications within them. Their topography is usually peripheral (Figure 9) (45).

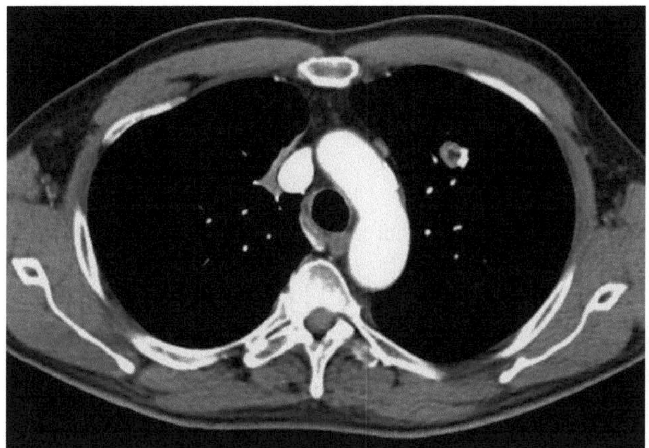

Figure 9: Hamartochondroma in the form of a nodule in the left upper lobe showing peripheral calcification and a central fatty component (45)

6.2. Lipomas

Lipomas are well-differentiated lesions, most often peripheral, with homogeneous fat attenuation on CT (45).. They are often diagnosed radiologically.

6.3. Endogenous lipid pneumonitis

Endogenous lipid pneumonitis is rare. Lipids accumulate in the alveoli as a result of upstream obstruction (carcinoma, bronchiolitis obliterans, pulmonary tissue necrosis following radiotherapy or chemotherapy), infection/chronic lung disease or a lipid storage disorder (46).

6.4. Bronchoalveolar carcinoma

The scannographic aspects of PLE can be observed in bronchopulmonary carcinomas (nodule, condensations, ground glass, crazy paving, etc.), which is why pathological examination is so important (47).

6.5. Pulmonary alveolar proteinoses

This is a rare disease characterised by the accumulation of surfactant components in the alveolus, which interferes with gas exchange.

The diagnosis is made on a chest CT scan in the presence of a Crazy paving appearance such as PLE (Figure 10). The diagnosis is based on the presence of PAS-positive lipoproteinaceous material on BAL in pulmonary alveolar proteinoses (48).

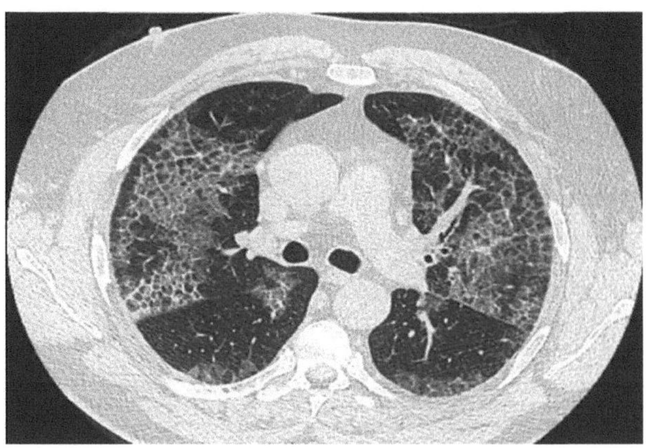

Figure 10: Diffuse crazy paving appearance in pulmonary alveolar proteinosis (48)

6.6. Infectious pneumonitis

More often than not, patients are treated as community-acquired infectious pneumonia, and another diagnosis is only considered when the patient does not respond to antibiotics because of the similar clinical and radiological picture (13).

6.7. Other

Crazy paving on CT can be seen in acute or chronic eosinophilic pneumonia, infections (Pneumocystis or Cytomegalovirus pneumonia), organised pneumonia and hypersensitivity pneumonia (2).

Treatment

7. Treatment

The treatment of exogenous lipid pneumonia is largely controversial, not well studied and the published literature contains only case reports.

7.1. Stop exposure

Avoidance of the offending product leads to improvement or even complete regression of the lesions within a few months. This depends on the extent and stage of the lesions (10).

Samhouri et al showed clinical and radiological deterioration despite stopping exposure because stopping exposure does not remove the previously aspirated material which initially provoked a foreign body type inflammatory reaction (12).

7.2. Corticosteroid therapy

Corticosteroid therapy has been considered effective in some cases (41, 49, 50). The effect of corticosteroids is to attenuate the body's inflammatory response to aspirated material.

However, corticosteroids are not always indicated and should only be used if the lung injury is severe (13).

However, the treatment regimen, including the compound, dose and duration, is not codified and the decision is team-dependent.

The treatment regimen, including the type, dose and duration of corticosteroid therapy, is not codified and the decision is team-dependent.

7.3. Therapeutic bronchioloalveolar lavage

Depending on the patient's condition, segmental bronchoalveolar lavage or whole-lung lavage may be performed.

The main mechanism behind the therapeutic effects of lung lavage could be its ability to eliminate aspirated substances, inflammatory factors caused by the body's immune responses and surfactants, which could interfere with normal gas exchange and trigger a process of pulmonary fibrosis (29).

In a review of the literature including 90 patients treated with bronchoalveolar lavage (alone or in combination with another treatment), 87 patients showed clinical improvement and 3 cases of in-hospital death (29).

7.4. Treatment of the contributing factor

Stopping the oily substance may not always be effective in patients who are often highly dependent on their treatment. If this is the case, treatment of a contributing factor such as anti-reflux therapy can at least limit inhalation of the oily substance.

7.5. Surgery

Surgery has little place in the treatment of lipid pneumonia. It is often indicated for diagnosis and may involve segmentectomy, lobectomy or wedge resection.

However, the diagnosis can be confirmed without recourse to invasive procedures by a good knowledge of the causes and manifestations of this condition, when the history, exposure, clinical, radiological and cytological findings are concordant (51).

Conclusion

Exogenous lipid pneumonias result from the penetration, usually by inhalation, of oily substances into the pulmonary parenchyma. These substances accumulate in the alveoli and pulmonary interstitium, either free or embedded in macrophages, and cause variable tissue reactions depending on the lipids involved.

The aim of this study is to examine the clinico-radiological presentations of lipid pneumonia and to define the diagnostic and therapeutic strategies.

Exogenous lipid pneumonia is a rare nosological entity. It is a disease of adults, the frequency of which increases with age.

Exogenous lipid pneumonia (ELP) can be acute or chronic. Acute ELP occurs when a large quantity of lipid substance is aspirated, whereas chronic exogenous lipoid pneumonia occurs after repeated episodes of aspiration or inhalation of lipids over a prolonged period.

In most cases, the lesions remain stable or slowly worsen, leading to impaired ventilatory function.

This study highlights the late and difficult diagnosis of PLE, due to a clinico-radiological presentation that is sometimes misleading in the absence of exposure.

A thorough history including possible exposures, including inhalation or aspiration of oily substances, helps to make the diagnosis of exogenous lipoid pneumonia.

Treatment remains uncoordinated. However, avoidance of exposure at an early stage is an effective treatment that can lead to regression or stability of lesions. Antibiotic treatment of bacterial superinfections may provide temporary relief of symptoms.

This underlines the importance of better knowledge and prevention to reduce the incidence of this condition and its impact on respiratory function.

References

References

1. Goenka U, Jajodia S, Jash D, Ghosh S, Bandyopadhyay S. Acute exogenous lipoid pneumonia: Unusual presentation as cavitating lung disease with pneumothorax. Respir Med Case Rep. 2022;36:101593.

2. Cozzi D, Bindi A, Cavigli E, Grosso AM, Luvarà S, Morelli N, et al. Exogenous lipoid pneumonia: when radiologist makes the difference. Radiol med. 2021;126(1):22-8.

3. Betancourt SL, Martinez-Jimenez S, Rossi SE, Truong MT, Carrillo J, Erasmus JJ. Lipoid Pneumonia: Spectrum of Clinical and Radiologic Manifestations. American Journal of Roentgenology. 2010;194(1):103-9.

4. Rea G, Perna F, Calabrese G, Molino A, Valente T, Vatrella A. Exogenous lipoid pneumonia (ELP): when radiologist makes the difference. Transl Med UniSa. 2016;14:64-8.

5. Marchiori E, Zanetti G, Mano CM, Hochhegger B. Exogenous lipoid pneumonia. Clinical and radiological manifestations. Respiratory Medicine. 2011;105(5):659-66.

6. Kuroyama M, Kagawa H, Kitada S, et al. Exogenous lipoid pneumonia caused by repeated sesame oil pulling: a report of two cases. BMC Pulm Med 2015; 15:135

7. Acharya V, Dsouza NV, Sreeram S, Rai SPV, Achappa B. Shine like gold and sparkle like glitter: Three cases of lipoid pneumonia. Respiratory Medicine Case Reports. 2021;33:101380.

8. Aliaga F, Chernilo S, Fernández C, Valenzuela H, Rodríguez JC, Aliaga F, et al. Exogenous lipoid pneumonia. Report of three cases. Revista médica de Chile. 2017;145(11):1495-9.

9. Gondouin A, Manzoni Ph, Ranfaing E, Brun J, Cadranel J, Sadoun D, et al. Exogenous lipid pneumonia: a retrospective multicentre study of 44 cases in France. European Respiratory Journal. 1996;9(7):1463-9.

10. Han C, Liu L, Du S, Mei J, Huang L, Chen M, et al. Investigation of rare chronic lipoid pneumonia associated with occupational exposure to paraffin aerosol. J Occup Health. 30 Sep 2016;58(5):482-8.

11. Osman GA, Ricci A, Terzo F, Falasca C, Giovagnoli MR, Bruno P, et al. Exogenous lipoid pneumonia induced by nasal decongestant. Clin Respir J. 2018;12(2):524-31.

12. Samhouri BF, Tandon YK, Hartman TE, Harada Y, Sekiguchi H, Yi ES, et al. Presenting Clinicoradiologic Features, Causes, and Clinical Course of Exogenous Lipoid Pneumonia in Adults. Chest. 2021;160(2):624-32.

13. Hadda V, Khilnani GC. Lipoid pneumonia: an overview. Expert Review of Respiratory Medicine. 2010; 4(6):799-807.

14. Doubková M, Doubek M, Moulis M, Skřičková J. Exogenous lipoid pneumonia caused by chronic improper use of baby body oil in adult patient. Revista Portuguesa de Pneumologia. 2013;19(5):233-6.

15. Nakashima S, Ishimatsu Y, Hara S, Kitaichi M, Kohno S. Exogenous Lipoid Pneumonia Successfully Treated With Bronchoscopic Segmental Lavage Therapy. Respir Care. 2015;60(1):e1-5.

16. Ohwada A, Yoshioka Y, Shimanuki Y, Mitani K, Kumasaka T, Dambara T, et al. Exogenous Lipoid Pneumonia Following Ingestion of Liquid Paraffin. Intern Med. 2002;41(6):483-6.

17. Le verre depoli : ses variantes et leur signification. Journal of Radiology. 2009;90(10):1441-2.

18. Choi HK, Park CM, Goo JM, Lee HJ. Pulmonary alveolar proteinosis versus exogenous lipoid pneumonia showing crazy-paving pattern: Comparison of their clinical features and high-resolution CT findings. Acta Radiol. 2010;51(4):407-12.

19. Harris K, Chalhoub M, Maroun R, Abi-Fadel F, Zhao F. Lipoid pneumonia: A challenging diagnosis. Heart & Lung. 2011; 40(6):580-4.

20. Yeung SHM, Rotin LE, Singh K, Wu R, Stanbrook MB. Exogenous lipoid pneumonia associated with oral and intranasal oil-based products. CMAJ. 2021 Dec 13;193(49):E1897-E1900. F

21. 0Marchiori E, Zanetti G, Mano CM, Irion KL, Daltro PA, Hochhegger B. Lipoid Pneumonia in 53 Patients After Aspiration of Mineral Oil: Comparison of High-Resolution Computed Tomography Findings in Adults and Children. Journal of Computer Assisted Tomography. 2010;34(1):9-12.

22. Chauveau R, Médart L, Ghaye B. Endogenous lipid pneumonia: a simple diagnosis? Rev Med Liege. 2005; 60(10): 799-804

23. Ukkola-Pons E, Weber-Donat G, Teriitehau C, Calcina P, Baccialone J, Vaylet F, et al. Imaging of oily pneumonitis. Feuillets de Radiologie. 2010;50(1):3-9.

24. Guo M, Liu J, Jiang B. Exogenous lipid pneumonia in old people caused by aspiration: Two case reports and literature review. Respir Med Case Rep. 2019;27:100850.

25. Khilnani G, Hadda V. Lipoid pneumonia: An uncommon entity. Indian J Med Sci. 2009;63(10):474.

26. Rana D, Kaushik N, Sadhu S, Kalra R, Sen R. Idiopathic Lipoid Pneumonia: An incidental finding in autopsy specimen. Autops Case Rep. 2020;10(1):e2020143

27. Wang Y, Goulart RA, Pantanowitz L. Oil red O staining in cytopathology. Diagnostic Cytopathology. 2011;39(4):272-3.

28. Basset-Léobon C, Lacoste-Collin L, Aziza J, Bes JC, Jozan S, Courtade-Saïdi M. Cut-off values and significance of Oil Red O-positive cells in bronchoalveolar lavage fluid. Cytopathology. 2010;21(4):245-50.

29. Shang L, Gu X, Du S, Wang Y, Cao B, Wang C, et al. The efficacy and safety of therapeutic lung lavage for exogenous lipoid pneumonia: A systematic review. Clin Respir J. 2021;15(2):134-46.

30. Jeelani HM, Sheikh MM, Sheikh B, Mahboob H, Bharat A. Exogenous Lipoid Pneumonia Complicated by Mineral Oil Aspiration in a Patient With Chronic Constipation: A Case Report and Review. Cureus. 2020;12(7):e9294

31. Maddock SD, Cirulis MM, Callahan SJ, Keenan LM, Pirozzi CS, Raman SM, et al. Pulmonary Lipid-Laden Macrophages and Vaping. N Engl J Med. 2019;381(15):1488-9.

32. Nielsen MH, Madsen LB, Bendstrup E. Exogenous lipoid pneumonia due to silent aspiration following surgery and radiotherapy for cancer of the tongue. Respir Med Case Rep. 2022;40:101767.

33. Pielaszkiewicz-Wydra M, Homola-Piekarska B, Szcześniak E, Ciołek-Zdun M, Fall A. Exogenous lipoid pneumonia - a case report of a fire-eater. Pol J Radiol. 2012;77(4):60-4.

34. Wong CF, Yan SW, Wong WM, Ho RSL. Exogenous lipoid pneumonia associated with oil pulling: Report of two cases. Monaldi Arch Chest Dis. 2018;88(3):922.

35. Rajagopala S, Selvam N. An unusual cause of respiratory distress. J Postgrad Med. 2019;65(1):38-40.

36. Ishimatsu K, Kamitani T, Matsuo Y, Hatakenaka M, Sunami S, Jinnouchi M, et al. Exogenous Lipoid Pneumonia Induced by Aspiration of Insecticide. Journal of Thoracic Imaging. 2012;27(1):W18-20.

37. Katsumi H, Tominaga M, Tajiri M, Shimizu S, Sakazaki Y, Kinoshita T, et al. A case of lipoid pneumonia caused by inhalation of vaporized paraffin from burning candles. Respiratory Medicine Case Reports. 2016;19:166-8.

38. Hotta T, Tsubata Y, Okimoto T, Hoshino T, Hamaguchi S, Isobe T. Exogenous lipoid pneumonia caused by herbicide inhalation. Respirology Case Reports. 2016;4(5):e00172.

39. Wangüemert Pérez AL. Neumonía lipoidea exógena secundario a uso de vaselina labial. Archivos de Bronconeumología. 2021;57(4):298.

40. García Latorre R, Rodríguez Díaz R, Barrios Barreto D, Ayala Carbonero A, García Gómez-Muriel MI, Gorospe Sarasúa L. Hallazgos radiológicos de la pneumonía lipoidea exógena en pacientes laringectomizados. Archivos de Bronconeumología. 2015;51(7):e36-9.

41. Park S, Park JE, Lee J. A case of lipoid pneumonia associated with occupational exposure to solvents in a dry-cleaning worker. Respirology Case Reports. 2021;9(6):e00762.

42. Gurell MN, Kottmann RM, Xu H, Sime PJ. Exogenous Lipoid Pneumonia: An Unexpected Complication of Substance Abuse. Ann Intern Med. 2008;149(5):364.

43. AlShamrani AS, Alzaid MA, Fadl SM, AlFaki MA. A case of infantile exogenous lipoid pneumonia with an unusual complication managed by modified whole lung lavage. Sudan J Paediatr. 2021;21(1):82-8.

44. Cherrez Ojeda I, Calderon JC, Guevara J, Cabrera D, Calero E, Cherrez A. Exogenous lipid pneumonia related to long-term use of Vicks VapoRub® by an adult patient: a case report. BMC Ear Nose Throat Disord. 2016;16(1):11.

45. Gaerte SC, Meyer CA, Winer-Muram HT, Tarver RD, Conces DJ. Fat-containing Lesions of the Chest. RadioGraphics. 2002;22(suppl_1):S61-78.

46. Gorra Al Nafouri M, Azar M, sbainy N, Al-bardan H. Idiopathic endogenous lipid pneumonia: A case report of a young Syrian man. Respir Med Case Rep. 2021;35:101547.

47. Da Costa FM, Cerezoli MT, Medeiros AK, Magalhães MAF, Castro SN. Small samples, big problems: lipoid pneumonia mimicking lung adenocarcinoma. J Bras Pneumol. 49(3):e20230147.

48. Jouneau S, Kerjouan M, Briens E, Lenormand JP, Meunier C, Letheulle J, et al. Pulmonary alveolar proteinosis. Revue des Maladies Respiratoires. 2014;31(10):975-91.

49. Alzghoul BN, Innabi A, Mukhtar F, Jantz MA. Rapid Resolution of Severe Vaping-induced Acute Lipoid Pneumonia after Corticosteroid Treatment. Am J Respir Crit Care Med. 2020;202(2):e32-3.

50. Lococo F, Cesario A, Porziella V, Mulè A, Petrone G, Margaritora S, et al. Idiopathic lipoid pneumonia successfully treated with prednisolone. Heart & Lung. 2012;41(2):184-7.

51. Chardin D, Nivaggioni G, Viau P, Butori C, Padovani B, Grangeaon C, et al. False positive 18FDG PET-CT results due to exogenous lipoid pneumonia secondary to oily drug inhalation. Medicine (Baltimore). 2017;96(22):e6889.

CONTENTS

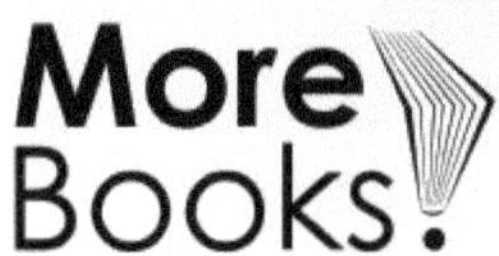

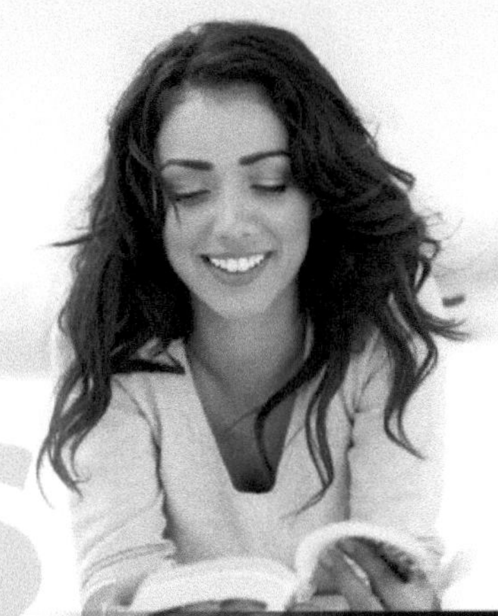

yes
I want morebooks!

Buy your books fast and straightforward online - at one of world's fastest growing online book stores! Environmentally sound due to Print-on-Demand technologies.

Buy your books online at
www.morebooks.shop

Kaufen Sie Ihre Bücher schnell und unkompliziert online – auf einer der am schnellsten wachsenden Buchhandelsplattformen weltweit! Dank Print-On-Demand umwelt- und ressourcenschonend produzi ert.

Bücher schneller online kaufen
www.morebooks.shop

info@omniscriptum.com
www.omniscriptum.com

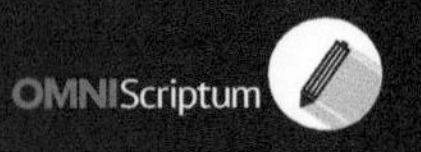

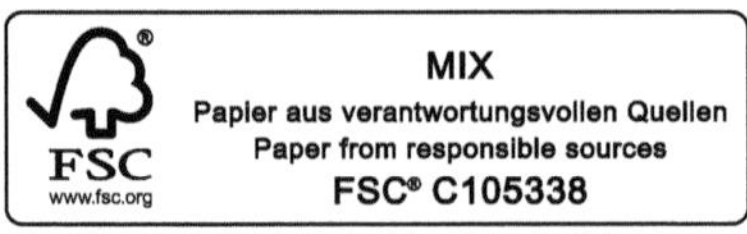

Printed by Books on Demand GmbH, Norderstedt / Germany